TRAUMA HEAD

Other books by Elee Kraljii Gardiner:

POETRY

serpentine loop

Trauma Head (chapbook)

ANTHOLOGIES

V6A: Writing from Vancouver's Downtown Eastside (co-editor)

Against Death: 35 Essays on Living (forthcoming)

TRAUMA HEAD

ELEE KRALJII GARDINER

anvil press • 2018

Anvil Press Publishers Inc.
P.O. Box 3008, Main Post Office
Vancouver, B.C. V6B 3X5 Canada
www.anvilpress.com

Library and Archives Canada Cataloguing in Publication

Gardiner, Elee Kraljii, 1970-, author
Trauma head / Elee Kraljii Gardiner. — First edition.

Poem.
ISBN 978-1-77214-122-1 (softcover)

I. Title.

PS8613.A743T73 2018 C811'.6 C2018-901891-7

Printed and bound in Canada
Edited for the press by angela rawlings
Cover design by Rayola Graphic
Cover photo by Alberto Seveso
Interior by HeimatHouse
Represented in Canada by Publishers Group Canada
Distributed by Raincoast Books

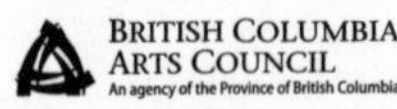

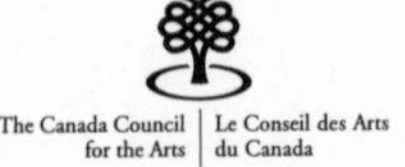

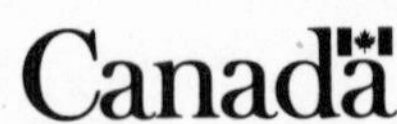

The publisher gratefully acknowledges the financial assistance of the Canada Council for the Arts, the Canada Book Fund, and the Province of British Columbia through the B.C. Arts Council and the Book Publishing Tax Credit.

Contents

I feel like a letter printed backward in the line.

– Søren Kierkegaard

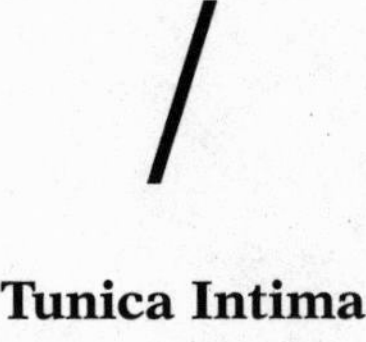

Tunica Intima

voices flashlight

where laughter is laser, clear-
cutting sleepiness

unbreakfasted, we are
here to work out-
side, repeat a schedule of health

field exhales
yesterday's heat
fogfoam above the grass

we runners scissor-
cut swathes
through this milk

none of us can
be sure where we stand

we see our bodies as flash,
reflective
vest, slurry of motion

in the witching we unspool
mats, swing weights

count, bend, crack

wise
about how tough we are

dew fastens
on keys dumped from pockets
chilled skin, bright euphoria
shoes veiled in diamonddrops

the body wakes
a market exchange of

conversion: blue to red

diaphanous fingerspread

all the vessels open to cells

the matrices, the uni-
ties
dawn written inside my eyelids

fogged breath, breathing fog

coyote swirl and still of owl

all the vesicles
surge
surf
miles of internal roads

o, adrenaline, my intimate!
o, endorphin, biologic morphine!

ventricles push and tumble, squeeze and
squeeze and receive – squeeze and receive – squeeze and receive

sugarcoaty synapses, superslick collisions
soundlessly oblivious

to the auricle, I

do not think
to brace myself
for tragedy in minuscule

butterfly effect across the network:
T minus seconds and

sit-up
if the left eyelid / twitch /
(sit-up)
if the left cheek / contract /
(-up)
if the forehead / prickle /
(-   )
if / the scalp / perfect delineation
left / right hemisphere

/ freeze

so cut the tongue in half
an ice travel down the arm
hand fist fall to mat
that tongue now the kettlebell

instant: lost / the clapper

/ mist /

now am soundless

/ how to call for help /

/ need

numb rush leftern to the centre line

the skull

I feel si where the brains don't meet
canyon gap

/

now
I'm in
the
vasse
/

snap fingers / slap / pound mat with some crumpled hand

kill their laughter
with a monster's voice
dull slab tongue

/ listen some / one

molasses legs un / zip

amphitheatre formation: 9 statues / 1 prone

switch: pulled

I know what this is. I won't say it, won't know it.

how tripped the wire

why fibre?

electrical disconnectal down leftside

erasure ~~of intention~~

silence along the left

. still

. meat

. blank where body has been

/ question-mined brain

am afraid

know where this is going

/

/

/

/

/

/

/

7 ½ minute / / ambulance

will never find in this dark

face up to stars
am newborn to danger

palm-sized
anchor
on my thigh
-ivering sets in

soon imperceptible slimslip
inside
slickening something refreshes, shunts
shakes free

nerves fizz / ig
nite
begin / speak / move

through a head spun
by systolic percussion and allegory

ETIOLOGY: Label all specimens with patient's first and last names, DOB and/or PHN & site. BODY: 3 TONGUE: <0 FOG: 3 SQUEEZE: 4 CUT: 2 BREATH: 0

she who I see as me

/ tiptoes back from woods /

black hound
bristles, charges
the 12-point stag, those ragged
antlers snagged oak

shocky, someone whispers

leftside afire, debris falling, architecture mid-bombing

who

is the

body

and how

quickly

tongue turns foreign

the body barbarian cask

some she sips mortal confusion

eyes full mooned

/ every instinct / geared to escape

/ *away*

from the body (the idea)

what has come
to dimidiate me

animalpanic and transformation
is now: I fable, I fate

sky carries cloud
curled brain has dropped
its load
of firewood
on the mirror pond

the forest I have to enter
a thicket a midnightfear

forced to duty / pushed to tunnel

coming, flags the ambulance

one step in and cannot see / surviving
within
tangles
of gorse

owls and wolves wait
for me to break
ferns, fallen limbs
catch my cloth, warn against rushing

she's / it's almost

moment s pin
lambswool longer-longer
Κλωθώ labours

slim digits tie knots to de-
ceive sister Ατροπος,
the scissor sister

spun, I nubble
mushrooms, dwarf apples, bitter greens,
touch spider sacs
and push fingertips into nurse logs

can you / are you

crows pull time / in ink trails / through silvered sky

bullet bodies sew themselves into precipitation,
contract time
whipstitch fear through heavens

I furl \ uncurl

furl / uncurl can I ?

a pair of signs: a field-grass bed, a stone pillow

night walks away, wordless

relinquishing the remainder
to a weak dawn service

and I am
suddenly thinking
about the barber

jars of bright blue comb juice

crisp part
drawn by black teeth

dividing left / right – everything
wrong

ɯıɹɹoɹ\ɹoɹɹıɯ

the carving
line is profound
needletight hemisphere

won't say it
though I've scanned the files:

/ stroke presents
/ fear aphasia - what will I w / out words –

/ yet I am think / placing yllables correct / am I not

catalogue simulacra: >ffwd
/ rehab / adaptive / / wheels
cyclical caregiving, drone

/ no / : alt del

no future of watchfulness

not this) again

will not adapt / ive

chip carve chisel dissever.   incise.

take the blade
by the knife

para / medic flash / light
iris sliver down beam
please deliver godtalk

what is your name?

/ L / E

how are you doing?

...

wordshell / jagged, familiar
impulse on tongue revolves
/ reveals blown-off face

when did it start?

...

what were you doing?

drop / thread...

Ατροπος *nearly* rouses

am ?
moving and touching ?
or words

flex ; wiggle

not / this / not this / ischemic event
: give them something else to read

syllab braid, twinning
circuit, hoop and ligature

uniforms ex
hort me

to slow

down
breath

pinned to mat I
run away

panting is hap
pening to me

like child
hood
redhead
edness / lefthand
edness

? I
leave

can't in / ex
past / stroke of 2

am cartoon cat
who left body behind
floating to a 9th
life fully formed

cat is 2 cats

cat is chalk outline

know / where I am
going / or for how long

I turn back
to the mat
which is empty

BODY:	5	TONGUE:	2	FOG:	0	AWAY:	3	CAT:	4	CUT:	2

medicine begins with losing a name
/
/
/
/
/
/
/
/
/
/
/
/
/
/
/
/
/
/
/
/
/
/
/
/
/
/ the bed is long and thin and hard and cold

pack animal: go where expected
crave curves, to burrow or nest
but recognize

cold and flat and thick and numb
am meant to be displayed

illness is platform
numb and cold and still and stiff
and this bed is built of violence

stiff and cold and thin and mute
brisk hands start a line
depart, return, withdraw, arrive

bring a blanket thin
as human skin

give body / over /
to whomever wants to touch it

in ter / en ter

scan pings
back upon itself
I sound /
the deep
recesses of the brain's fjords, too
I want / to
navigate by familiar
buoy of pain

but all I sense is mist

and every shadow

here, have it, I'll unfold
miles of myself into capable hands
unspool veins and empty all my arteries
within the pages of the chart

unfold / become
lotus in heat

flutter and bloom on this bed

opening (dilating ((

read me how you like
me / an instrument
prized for pliability, unobstructionist
and unmysterious

I'll make it easy
pull shirt off shoulder
push palms
into your capable hands
wait for you to decide
if I am as strong as I appear

the door swings

valve / view: chairwheeled man
grips his head

2 coatholders staff his shoulder, silent archangels

door swings again

he is on bed

eyes closed

i.v. / an empty thought bubble

and the angels are gone

in / ter / im
in the e-room, in-
terminable
I'm
a / lone, i / solated / solo

appearance: Robert fills the door
the scent of his neck
carries mudhoneycalm

he scrutinizes, reconciles
she fainted
with what he sees / hears
so normal: exercise clothes, ruffled ponytail
an ability, a joke
cheeks roughed pink

/ did not faint: the stain
in the glass is darker
taint is swirling
nothing is settled

give me your hand, I pant
he sits starboardside
where he cannot see
my lines are cut

and vessels are drifting to wreckage

he, relaxing

he thinks I look just fine

he thinks I look just fine

/ I meet my body from the inside

twitch of a fin
flex of the spine:
am become animal

a goose flown off / course

anthropomorphize me, I beg
the resident who advises
as an afterthought

make sure to keep your head above your heart

stunned dumb
unable
to question
the kill bolt

rapid insufflation
chimes
the room

the resident already departs

rows of tests to follow or / or / or

run / the tongue /

touched, unfolding

I *look ok*

I am

offline

walking to the car
slow as the stalked – or am ? hunter –

; unflex tingled hand
fiddle / crab
lifted from sand, grasping air
I / run / the tongue /
touch / parts of my body
with its correspondent

half of me
believes I am ok
(I sound, think, talk)
other me is dumb

he opens the bottle
drops a seed
on muscle

all the way home I test residue

HANDS: 5 BODY: 3 BED: 4 TONGUE: 2 UNFOLD: 2 SILENT: 1 COLD: 4

return

the house pauses when I enter / shifts /
windowpanes fleer, carpet fibers wilt under my feet
couch cushions exhale
their suspicions

the dieffenbachia is snide
about my unsteadiness

I taste malevolence in the air

or is it burnt toast?
he is cracking
eggs because there's nothing
a hot meal can't fix

can't lie down / count down
ticking
inside head
deadline

pulse beat thrum / pulse beats thrum / pulses beats thrums /

¡ ping !

? short circuit is / be now ¿

cat jumps
I flinch

he drops a fork
ricochet for 15 minutes
inside

room crowds
with crows / strobes

an orchestra of confusion sawing
away
run (

when
do you
need
anything right now

is to hand-sew finest stitches
on a torn seatbelt on the Tilt-A-Whirl

// nap of pillow
comes at me
with a megaphone

// his podcast
from the other room
is a wave of razors

run (

moment to moment the bubble
in the spirit level

pared of street clothes, rules / duties
an axis of capacity shifts

the children know
all they want
to know: the inside
of the ambulance that took me
from the park at 6:20 a.m. on September 20
in the dark through the fog

had a bed, a chair, a bench
cubbies for supplies

a cunning boat

siren left unlit

through the cornfields
of blacked-out farm towns
where ozone singes neurons
the cattle face the rain

an internal cycle

/ is gathering / is a there ring / at the ring / weathering

cells thrown, thrown
switched
crown
the crow
dips
down

the first panic approaches
/ siren

second panic
couples
fine-tipped awareness
nothing is natural
not how move / am breathe / a think
am foreigner to myself
immigrating to shores of fear

I pack a wet idea in a cardboard suitcase:
miles of headaches
body can't
withstand more
than 5 minutes of this

it will quit / it doesn't

thirdfourthfifth panic attack: longer /

can't / keep body

still

writhe and fidget / wridget and fithe

cat pads away

don't / know go
where safe /
familiar
loaded
threat

in the sweetness
of the children's rooms
beds / abandoned, tousled / signal: intruder on premises

I invigilate floorboards
examine window locks
on my frame of mind, rattle
bars on the house
of language

enter the disruption /

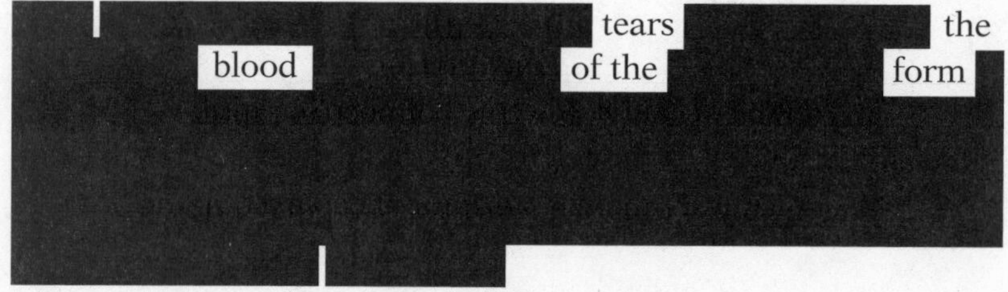

enter the disruption /

Petals of the many-sided tree and inside corners arise from tears that occur in the broken layer, allowing blood under flatline pressure to enter the wall of the vessel and form a tinted glass. Disruption of the jellyroll can activate maps and the cornered cascade, leading to wall formation and bright silver.

enter the disruption /

Wives of the orange and colourful people
arise from tears that occur in the disquiet layer
allowing blood under substantial pressure to enter the wall
of the vessel and form blissful sleep
disruption of the. Water can activate
children and the radiant cascade
leading to swan formation and silky rain

enter the disruption /

horses of the Finnish
heredity and fluorescent.
Dendrites arise from tears
that occur in the delicate layer, allowing blood
under indelicate pressure
to enter the wall
of the vessel and form
a Flemish candour.
Disruption of the heiress can activate whores
and the worst cascade, leading to source formation
and feverish hordes.

enter the disruption /

flummoxed by stiffen these creeps miles
hang pepperpots don't I or
do
catch that river schist in crickets
and slyly die

enter the disruption /

assassin smells
cinched in to be crisped ‘n’ crinkled
whole carps in lugubrious gong show

sludge holder is cryful
cripsy scrimps crammed in kilos

enter the disruption /

allow lonely bloodache

a loll on calendar

deal, fever-freak

ease eludes squeamy

flee, elee

shut //

sleeping is braincomicstrip
braindance hypercolourplay
unconfined neural rollercoaster
kickracing away from the barn

twenty minutes dims
the buzz constant tenant
upstairs is quieter after re / set
burning of left side tames

the world is slightly softer
as the horses nose back to the barn

little infauna, I am
rooted in the benthic zone
feeding on scraps of touch and breath
wrecked

bury books in sand
/ part burial, part safe-keeping /
they may be salt-chewed and soaked
before my return, if a return,

if -

struggle to hold / *if* / just so
in the cup of my ear
delicately
as a branch of fire coral in my palm

stung
I surge, become *cenote*
steamhole, sourspout

BLOOD: 3 BODY: 5 BED: 2 PULSES: 4 BREATH: 2 TEARS: 3

cannot a body is glass

cannot see through it
yet
here peer
into mirror of belly, doubled
with apprehension

lumen, window, ill lumen

there is a true and false lumen

cannot pick up
fragments

cannot bend
cannot recover
a dropped —

must keep *head above heart*
where it has never ruled
must think before
cannot re / act

the carpet studded and littered
with lost gerunds:

redesign

vocabulary hauls antenna higher
verbs n / either serve
n / or appreciate my hard work
selecting them

meaning boils over
a telephone call burns the pan dry

leftside
obtund, draped films
tamp skin on ½ face and L. arm

sun
numbed / fire
sided

or was worked too hard, muscles unreliabled

electrical shocks matrix under skin

/ fearritated /

word will match word

if / eyes can take it or / ears can: / not both /

enter soundscapes
verboten for too janglecrimping

precipitant
puttied hands
unbraid tangled
veins of tinsel

only sitting
quietly
in front of a bowl of thought

Vertebral artery dissection (VAD) is one of the most common identifiable **I turn face to pillow** causes of stroke in those aged 18-45, with an estimated annual incidence between 1 and 1.5 per 100,000. Since VAD is a potentially treatable cause of transient ischemic attack (TIA) and stroke, and the greatest risk of stroke in craniocervical **blunt the bright** dissections appears to occur in the first few weeks after dissection, prompt diagnosis is essential. **ness of the world** Unfortunately, VAD is not always easily recognized, and young patients with missed VAD may suffer potentially disastrous neurologic complications or death. Frank presentations of stroke, TIA, or subarachnoid hemorrhage (SAH) are likely to initiate an inpatient hospitalization and complete diagnostic workup, including vascular imaging, but **can't understand** patients with VAD may present with nonspecific complaints such as dizziness with neck pain, or headache **what you are** with nausea and vomiting. Although VAD is more likely to be considered in patients with a clear history **saying** of trauma or with known underlying connective tissue disease, in some cases **again** neither of these known risk factors is present. The literature describing VAD is varying in quality **again** and content, and many studies report on only a few crystalline patients. The purpose of this study was to conduct a systematic review of studies reporting clinical and **skidding** radiographic data **along miles**, on individuals with VAD, to determine both the level of evidence available on this topic and to identify core clinical features of the syndrome. We sought to characterize the frequency **shrewd routes** of various symptoms, ischemic complications, and spectrum of outcomes in individuals with **studded with** VAD. **campaniles**.

the clot, the block
the body on strike

neurologist
is on the line

a tear in the endothelium
the skin, eggshell membrane
torn away in the artery in the neck

endothelium: funereal word for specialized tissue

a type of *epithelium*, the connective fabric
lining the interior
of this coffin

a *tunica intima*
the innermost lining

and behind the diagnosis
of a rent in the veil
is a deeper plot
sleeper cells
thickandthicker
upon themselves
in a viscid nest

the slit in the nightgown
was but symptom
of commination
sliding down the brain stem

mistake this linen
for *epithalamium,* a poem
written for a bride
en route to the marriage bed
to her own *petite mort,* if luck
is moonsoaked

he speaks *intimal flap*
rip in the shroud, 3.2 cm

: same length
as the pterodactyl's wingspan
on the children's ruler

palpate bony ladder to skull
with dumb fingers /senseless /

run (future tense: the doctor and I
view film footage
of this artery of mine together

) *intima*
(he recognizes parts of me
I have never seen myself

dr. describes a sheaf, a rip, thinnest
membrane peeled from wall

/ water blistering paint /

double lumen in the vertebral artery

there is a true and false lumen

salve, epithelium! salute
nomenclature

complicated names are better than none

no insult

neither trauma nor torque

nor crash suggests why

) typical dissection headache which *may / may not* resolve

the tear in the fabric, hole in a pocket
may / may not mend itself
via dissevered weeks

and I *may / may not* experience spontaneous —
) keep an I out

may be some months before
maybe earlier cells bred clot
infixed in brain stem

>>>> blew free fast as spitball through straw >>>>

the only medicine proffered is the tincture of time

) they science around but resolve little

xi so flew non the door
fieth on arc

so why am I staring

hey / am on del / ay
have come / blin / king from a diet / ary cave of stro / be lights
and vid / eo games, speed / metal play / ed at high volume

you asking
someth – ing
/ solve-ish complex algebraic equation faster, FASTER
or maybe

you said hello

in the middle of the

night, awoked and alaughed
some mild dreamline
sets a riot inside

with / in moments am lost
in laughter, awoken him
careen from laugh / her to laugh / to / tears
body reads laugh / = / threat
heated / threatened
soblaugh, sweat tears from nape to leg pits
cheeks swashed and heat throwing reflex at the ceiling
cannot stop the force of feeling

no difference
to my body between safe and scare

and it is this
realization that makes
me feel
unhinged

I learn *labile*

learn causes or roots
learn patience — wait
learn *limit*

mid-conversation burst
and blubber

reasonless
emotionswath

body betrayer turn mindelectrical, unpredicatable
dicto, dictare,
mirabile dictu (*non*)
no (w) body is an onlytruth
now body is the crave
ownlanguage

bodytouch
it all
and
I don't
ask before
touching
you

con / fusion

I leave the house
once a day if
I have to

the little one says
my *temper span*
has shortened

spontaneous vertebral artery dissection

twisting through the copse
of strangers' stories
I have 20 mins of straightthought
for a field of narratives
that circle back to loss

meat-eating beast
at the heart of the maze
I'm afraid / will have to bivouac here
then discover a clause / a clearing
a picnic pre-arranged, spread
over uneven stony ground

a quartet of northern cardinals
alights beside me
I stay statue
do not wish to disturb the aleatory
forces at work
this stroke of good

balanced on the teeth of the comb
tighten my little bird claws
on slimmest lines

:
:
:
:
:
:
:
:
:
:
:
:
:
:

:
:
:
:
:
:
:
:
:

:
:

:
:
:
:
:
:
:
:
:
:
:
:
:
:
:
: colour of cushion
: weight of blanket
: wind in chimney
: chafe upon ankle
: molar against tongue
: wind in ears
: electric noise coursing house
: surge of current
: throb in hear
: pulse in throat
: tinderbells in eustachia
: bright ice of light
: cut of cold in tiles
: tin of sound
: knotted at the ends, they clump

won't pull through

paltry hunger for thought
is damped
by Sisyphean registration
of mundane components

inside the brain
pathways reroute

feel them run (

my body
is runbody, fearbody
I have miles of headaches
everyday miles of headaches
I cannot run miles headaches
miles of headaches miles of
headaches miles of headaches pain
walks miles of headaches miles of
fearaches miles of headaches miles of
headaches miles of heartaches miles
of heart I cannot start miles of
headaches miles of headaches miles
of headaches miles of headaches I
cannot run heart cannot run miles of
headaches miles of headaches miles
of headaches miles of headaches
miles of headaches of headaches of
headaches of aches

................inside
..........................autumn

grey

.......................body............

...........forgets............................

...............word

....for.....

.....moving

cancel

show no
inclination of tiring
couched / pajamaed / abed

feel my way past mirrors, purblind
to the idea of reflection

discrepancy between placid image outside
and jumbledness within
irreconcilable

so, lassitude.

He suggests
dinner out

cannot / formulate form / carve response

heave away, squalling

leftsideface slid downsome
clothbound abed

joyless instruct
to children
keep hands
away from my neck

transparence re: illness – no effort

they see through the pane

I am a double of what I was

dull and closed

I false lumen

HEADACHES: 195 BODY: 8 FOG: 0 TEARS: 5 LUMEN: 4 HANDS: 2 SILENT: <0

I do not care for anything.
I do not care to ride
for the exercise is too violent. I do not care
to walk, walking is too strenuous.
I do not care to lie down, for I should either
have to remain lying, and I do not care to do that,
or I should have to get up again, and I do not care to do that either.
Summa summarum: I do not care at all.

— Søren Kierkegaard

trick: shut

: reducing what comes in
buys minutes
of function

in morning am spat out
of surf
lashed with cold threads

remove bullkelp strands

1 by 1

strip down to skeleton impulse

pretendless

the tongue roams

daylight's 81mg

a feather-weight act
of prevention

no other treatment
so choose belief

again the taste of childhood

this unknowing

the distance between

myselves

a typography of—

the kerning between—

rive, riven:

such hurried and violent rush

distance between myselves: 3.2 cm
distance measurable in grained frames

mete: the length of a safety pin
joint of index
electrical outlet mouth

/ so test / click
photo after photo
the cold eye captures
portraiture of halves

me mimic Richter
squeegeesmear paintings

/ grey /: storm-smeared left
the other side composed, untouched /

facefall,
selfdropped

couldn’t motherboard
synapse shortout

happen / now?

dis / ability—mortality—this flip
unhandled switch

\ brainslip is glass

and the world is
pouring, pouring

an endless stream

crouch, wince, would
run (

if only it were safe
to jar the vessel

lying next to littler bodies
fear swipes in

am thinking / what if I miss / am un / able to –
until fear also burns out under the buzzer

rasp of leg against a sheet
a schoolyard story

every moment
is inside crowding
brainpain input shoutSHOUTs

openmouthed language caesura / use
little's metronomic breath to pace

decipherish the syntax
of the heated body

am alligator mind
tasting

relearn the word
by tonguing
world

on the only
event, a drive to school
measure
clear space / counting
the spin of interior odometers

attent: *subito* sting
hands turn blunt
assume fight for normal
panic anesthetizes / right

/ or should pull over is this the big 1 /

in back the children natter, ask for a radio change
they freeze when snap

hear my body
better through their silence?

children kiss me softly, my apology
in their pockets
a flesh-ripped fruit, leaking

distance from school to home:
11 minutes—a continent

hazards on, I call Robert
he steps me through the door
his voice low velvet

nap resects funhouse dreams

fall into the disruption
snuggies of the ambivalent pierogi and garish
hipsters arise from tears that occur in the dinky layer
allowing blood under churlish pressure
to enter the wall of the vessel and form
a bourgeois underdog
disruption of the zipper can activate mosquitoes
and the smarmy cascade, leading to blackguard
formation and profound platitude

brain cavorts
stretching and playing
jokes behind my back

memory and thought
are actors on stage
in the frontal cortex

this haywire / live action sleep show
is skit-based: brain conversing with itself

when I rise
the twitch is left behind
somewhere I don't remember
an arterial thrum

rises / pressure building / I stay still

BODY: 3 COLD: 2 TONGUE: 2 BRAIN: 2 VESSEL: 2 CARE: 7

crop:

haircutter knows something
happened, measures 3 months

he reads growth
first white hair is trauma
a jettison

body, are you honest?

time unspools its white thread
constant proof am altered

crop:

haircutter knows something
happened, measures 3 months

he reads growth
first white hair is trauma
a jettison

body, are you honest?

time unspools its white thread
constant proof am altered

I crumple
sheets
of aluminum

foil into a Viking hat
become less fritzed,

joke hat repels
wayward painbeams
from outlets, from aliens

littlest one
finds me tearing up
tortured by sandfleas and greenheads
caught in brainfolds

he runs for hat

here, Mama, here

soundhammer taps
on the keystone of the arch

and I, old edifice, buckle

he is millstone's circle

he folds back almost-clean sheets
in the shape of calm

navigates tidetables

scarcely
remarks how schismatic
the form on the floor is

how wifelike I
am not above the flatline

breeze motion colour sound balance:
the walk costs me an hour's sleep

armed
with material
an empty road
pitted / panic /
pop-up target practice
in the heart's alley
no one
sees me
going down

riot night of tinnitus
I wake from the drill in the ear

reading is recorded / I won't watch footage

feel the fact of dis / section in the constant headache
yearlong / er
someone mentions
speaking rather slowly
neuro-opthamologists confer

pupils di / late / contract at differing speeds

bifurcated woman, halved, seamed, I am studied

we wait

continued studies

another port, this one

opened

to a bag of rad / io / actives
hung off the machine

hot particles slide
translucent into the tide
face blooms an ochre sweat
and bitter almond dampens my palms

my beaches turn calescent
the floating dock
stormtossed

dreamed I could
jump
out an airplane
above
an unfolded city / if /
I presented passport, money and *jumping* shoes

sorrow: missed a beautiful chance
because could not organize
3 simple things

he moves his palm along my thigh
and I snap

every millimetre of skin
demands deciphering billions
of messages

am backlogged with info of my own
pinging against overloaded circuit board

be simple, be

leave your hand there
as long as you don't move

morning unhemmed

torned

I hear him sluicing dipthongs across paper

a leaf drops syllables from the potted plant

rain spits at the window in a foreign language

I am aware
I am waning

a consumptive *tsarina*
melancholy chords
melodrama: how useless this is

love, I call
can you please bring me a cookie
because I've had a stroke, you know

ink in ill / able

BODY: 1 HEADACHE: 1 STUDY: 3 UNCHANGED: 2 WHITE: 2 DISSECTION: 3

magnets bid metal

healer digs fingers in my scalp
draws away
at the end of each stroke
flicks invisible ribbons
she likens to black licorice laces

do I believe?

as plausible as God
or neurologist

her idea
incorporates,
at least, touch

she serves a glass of water
observes, enjoins me
to take to the loam
the forest, somegoodmud
somelement of grounding
a pineneedle walk over horse manure
culverts and coyote trails
antidotes to electric revenge

truth: all I crave is touch and yes it is

dirt and iodine
of beach morning drizzle
        wetbloom smell in wind
make me heady

                all dogs catch oceanspritz in their coats

                                flash / to the other side of this stroke
        memory jog / remember /
                                racing men
                                at the park, accelerating past them

try
a few / steps
but pain flies
roosts behind left eye

                pull up / lame

burst into tears amidst sand
fend off a cluster of puppies

        the world won't let me go / keeps pulling me
                                                forward into beauty

I want to touch
want heavy cells
soaked with deep breath
want to warm my hand on the nape
to settle leg upon leg, slide it, slurring
like a bow, legato, elongated
want his voice moving through
my ribcage
code to heart muscle
I lean into the shoulder
            siphon, charge

she walks me
adjusts
/ slow gaited /
she catches me wordless

across the continent sister says
once she sees
me she'll know
I'm alright

/ alone / I
notice bright
twisting, leaves
fall into
terrifying colour

blood drains out the lethal frame

calculus of risk: add up percentage points hyperlinked to the body

it will take practice
but she will learn my dissimilar speed
bring me tea / sit

when I cup hands in my lap
nest them like empty eggshells

whites of my eyes bared

both of us waiting

choose / laugh /
drive up the mortal hill
grinding the teeth
of gears, trusting the gas gauge
flickering past orange has it wrong

make it on fumes
heartbeat
traipses behind

mats like cells
populate the dim room
my body re / members first pose / child's pose

) hisses) *keep your head above your heart*

upwelling, something dissolving
sinkingidon'tevenknowwhat
glassed pane
can't stop / tears rebounding on solar plexus
packeddownclot of 5 months' fear
stone of not moving

corpse pose strikes close / I lose
somewhere behind me another woman sobs

this room is grief

/ or loss
/ or relief

names are unimportant now

slice
the dissolving mass
with a wobbly hand
I bisect
some clotted idea, expecting the pellucid
wet heart of identity

the sadness of the work surprises

saw until I'm in 3rds
sloppily spilt into brain
as organ / soul / mind

piles drawl
decisive pumpkin guts

hollowed, I can't decide
if *feelings* belong to brain or mind
and does *pain* partition to brain or body?

never thought of brain as muscle
until it spoke as independent limb

) how it heats in the MRI microwaving
pulsing me with dizziness

who has dominion?
and is mind affected by brain's injury
and if it is, where is self
and can it define *scathed*?

no, no, do not trust the instrument

silence, rain
keeps me in

quiets the folds of rumpled grey matter
life has begun to dangle its demands
urging me to unlock unused rooms

I spend my 20 minutes
revising an excerpt of a memoir on trauma

touching someone else's words
about before / after
reminds me:
how swiftly we / are al / tered
all of us re / novated
by exposure to pain and
what we cannot control

somewhere in memory
a boulder drops into a quarry reservoir

the plummet and splash
perversely pleasing
because the body does not surface

pain wears me

is the tide
chewing cliff face
pain wears me

this injury tumbles me in the chop
is the tide

chewing cliff face
any hiatus pain wears me

in the repetition of panic
this injury tumbles me in the chop
is the tide

left gleaming and new chewing cliff face
pain wears me
any hiatus
polished through abrasion
in the repetition of panic
this injury tumbles me in the chop
is the tide

chewing cliff face
left gleaming and new
any hiatus
polished through abrasion
in the repetition of panic
this injury tumbles me in the chop

left gleaming and new
any hiatus
polished through abrasion
in the repetition of panic

left gleaming and new
polished through abrasion

when basaltic glass cracks
the syringe pulls in

I feel the lace
of steel through tissue

glissade epinephrine-enhanced delivery
legs want to pump, flee
from deepnumb spreading
to thoughts of the last minute / before /

mirror symptoms
/ again / on my back, mouth useless
under the lamp
hands
clumsy moths

people slip
out of the room, leave
me / collect / myself
like something lost

I plunge blue
and the tongue lolls
down the fjord walls of dreamtime

a shiny veneer
removed

under it is something struggling, some thing bent
on enunciation

the body is the bag that needs things

BODY:	6	BREATH:	3	TURN:	3	FOG:	2	LINE:	3
TOUCH:	2	FEELING:	6	FEAR:	2	HANDS:	2	HEAD:	3

sailing through
the flea market

life's wreckage
breaks
over flotsam

a man jumps in front of me
screaming *fuck you! fuck off!*

then grapples someone into a bear hug

the held man
bursts out
laughing and the 2
separate and fist bump

I haul in, tighten
the jib, navigate away
before I collapse in myself

everything scares me—the flutter of gills
around me, the *ticktick* of breaking
coral fathoms below

want to uncoil
thoughts but my hands are brittle
horseshoe crabs kicked up to the wrack line

a friendly man brings to my table
a cup of coffee and a wreath of risk

he sits expectant, repeats questions, taps
every clink of his spoon / unsafe /

light flickers through the sharp window
bitter chatter register coffee grinder screams

I cannot find a moment to connect
do not want connection

/ so who am I now /

when spring infection settles
I cough up starlight splinters
retinal patterns pinprick
          the eastern seaboard
                    of my brain

each hack hooks
                    an anchor claw
          inside my brainsoftshell
                                        draws me along the seabed to
                                                  the lip of the trench

a cough could crack me
clot me again

I tunnel under to join
a population
hiding fear / paranoia / panic

I know only the corner
of this territory, I know

I merely squat here
while some are its fat kings

she imagines pain, touches
her neck as I speak
          how terrifying she asks without upswing

the body demands definitions, so many / so much
                                                                  narrative

the neurologist stops returning / my calls :   I must
                                                                      be better

at least you can play the s-card
she says, flashing
the c-card she got for cancer
meet you at the front of the line!

have I invented
exaggerated / prolonged
called forth /created /desired or
designed this?
crossed the line between
psycho /somatic

in / soma
/ situ
/ side
/ sincere
/ significant

when the headache stops
a year to the day
I turn around to look for it

only the clock spins until the wave hits

every surface is made of wood
watch how I rap the sturdy gunwale

cleared

permitted to pick
a button from the floor
allowed to drop
my head
          and reassert the heart's dominion

                    encouraged to return
                              though the park makes me swirl—
                                        a graveyard with / out bodies; jinxed

the pounding and thrumming thrushpath
of blood in my ears is so recently shushed
                    I prefer to slip into the pool, a gentler
          daytime of elders on spindle sticks
neurodiverse teens with rolling eyes
          see-through lycra stretched over mountains
          mole-stamped freakiness of the general public

the man treading next to me in the dive pool
          passes required minutes
          relating the habit that wrecked him
          and the spinal cord injury that corrected
          a corkscrewed life

          a year:
          I have been
          cleared

white-haired nonna
body a bag of flour
hoists up the diving board stairs
pshaws the Chinese man with whom she shares
only swimlanguage
they are puppyish, silly, loudmouths, flirtful

she breaches like an orca, magnificent and heavy
and we roar for our lady
applause shakes droplets from our hands

seniors recognize me through quotidian
nods and thumbs up
they decipher my envy, use eyebrows
to urge me up
no is not allowed, I know
the year of safety concussed my *anima*

I walk the thin rib of plank
and bounce back into a space before the fear
/ backwards
flipping d / ang / er to ang / le

up and over re / volving re / viving

I break
the surface, burst
forth re / known to myself, I high
five the woman in the bathing cap

reel in cheers
cut the belly of fear wide
slide in, rehouse, reinhabit myself

cell upon cell
strength returns
the softened body might muscle

the lungs refill with less huff
beyond the body I am changed
into an object convinced of its own
impermanence

by my shoulder is a shadow even on brightest solstice
an *always*
some noonday dot ready to dilate

terror swoops and deletes, bathes me in dread
retreats by degrees too minimal to measure

daily inoculation: recession

perhaps revival will stick

my left side trembles, in case I forget

under the skin
the lining, a warning true and false

/

Trauma Head File

NOTE: This is information at a point in time and updates/addendums may not be fully reflected on printed copies. The report should be revised again online to ensure the most current information is used before making clinical treatment decisions.

SEP 2 6 2012 Vancouver CoastalHealth

Promoting wellness. Ensuring care.

MEDICAL IMAGING REQUISITION

FAXED SEP 2 7 2012

☐ X-Ray ☐ CT ☐ Ultrasound ☐ Echo ☐ Angiogram/Interventional ☐ Nuclear Medicine

Any Site ☐ or Specify Site: ____________ Appointment Date: ____________ Time: ______

PATIENT

PHN ____________ ICBC ____________

PHN: [redacted] MRN: [redacted]
[redacted], ELEE
2[redacted]70 41 F
VANCOUVER BC IFD: N
D:(604)[redacted] N:(604)[redacted]

PHN: [redacted] MRN: [redacted]
[redacted] ELEE
22Dec1970 41 F
ACCT: [redacted] SV NEU Acct End Date: 19Sep13
BENAVENTE, OSCAR(MD)
LOCATION: Stroke Prevention IFD: N

Tel: ____________ Other: ____________

Date of Birth: ____ ____ ____ M☐ F☐

Previous Images? Location: ____________

Escort Required ☐ Nurse ☐ Porter ☐ Volunteer

Mode of transport ☐ Wheelchair ☐ Stretcher ☐ Bed

Other ☐ O_2 ☐ Isolation ☐ Portable ☐ IV Pump

DOCTORS TO COMPLETE THIS SECTION

EXAM(s) REQUESTED:

CTA × arch to vertex

Physician should consult with Radiologist for Urgent and Stat cases

Priority
☐ Routine
☒ Urgent
☐ Stat

Able to give consent? ☐ Yes ☐ No If the patient does not speak English, an interpreter **MUST** accompany the patient

Pt diabetic ☐ Yes ☐ No
On metformin ☐ Yes ☐ No
Breast Feeding ☐ Yes ☐ No
Pregnant ☐ Yes ☐ No
LMP ______
G ____ P ____ A ____
Height ______ Weight ______
Previous contrast reaction?

PERTINENT HISTORY / MEDICATIONS:

URGENT!

TIA - ?? Right temporal

Physician's signature [redacted] Tel: Physician's MSP billing #: [redacted]

Copies of report to: [redacted]

This section MUST be completed if requesting CT

Is Kidney Function abnormal? ☐ Yes ☐ No Has patient had L-spine surgery? ☐ Yes ☐ No

If YES for any of the above OR if requesting a CT Abdomen/Pelvis OR Angiogram: a current (within 3 months) eGFR and Creatinine are mandatory:

eGFR: 73 Date: Sept 20 - 2012

Creatinine: 76 Date: Sept 20 - 2012

This section MUST be completed for all Core Biopsies, Angiograms and Interventional Procedures

INR: ______ Date: ______ * Does the patient take anticoagulant/anti-platelet medication? ☐ Yes ☐ No

PLATELETS: ______ Date: ______ If yes please list medications:

eGFR: ______ Date: ______

Creatinine: ______ Date: ______

*Patients may have to stop taking anticoagulant or anti-platelet medication prior to their appointment. If this is unsafe for your patient please consult a radiologist.

DEPARTMENT USE

Technologist: ______
Date: ______
No. of Images: ______
Fluoro Time/Dose: ____ / ____
Shielding used: ______
Technologist comments on reverse

hospital complex

cold fat in steam

one eye / left eye

small smaller slow

00083312, VCH.0026 June 2010

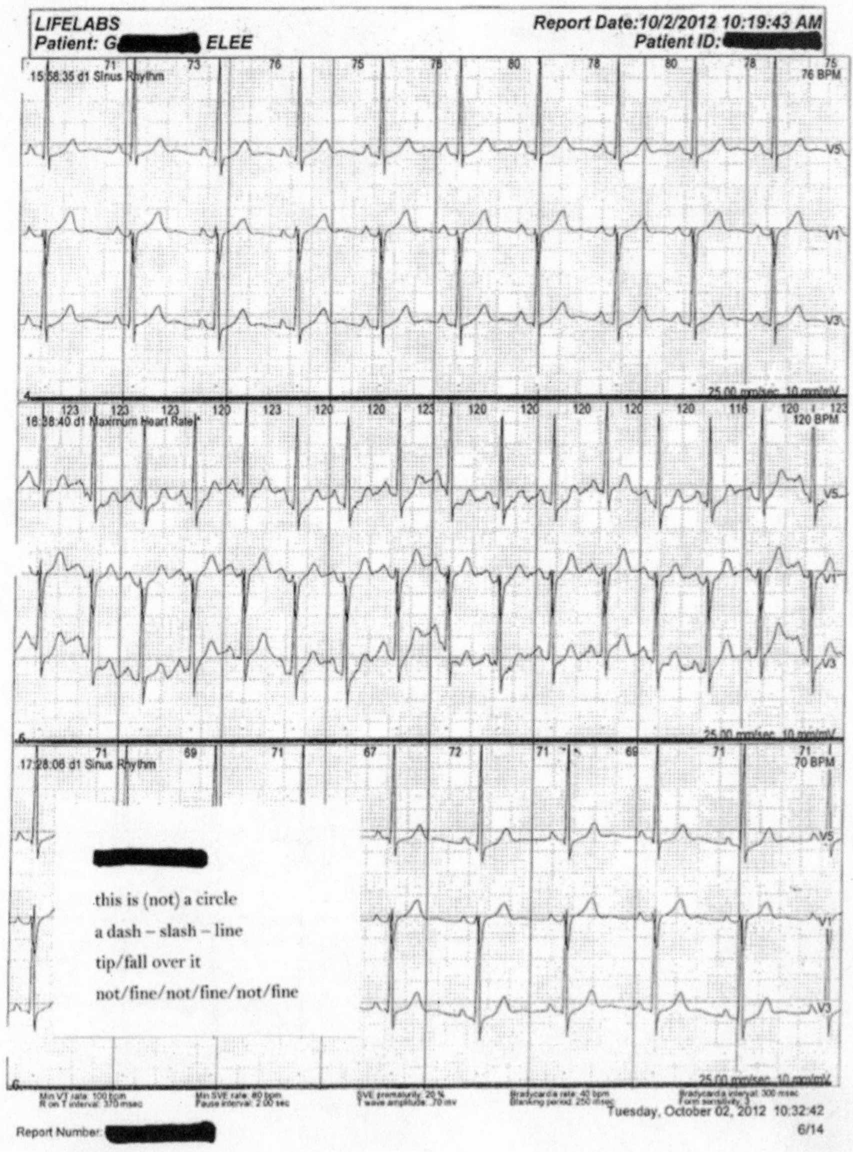

LIFELABS
Patient: G[redacted] ELEE

Report Date:10/2/2012 10:19:43 AM
Patient ID:

15:58:35 d1 Sinus Rhythm — 76 BPM

16:38:40 d1 Maximum Heart Rate* — 120 BPM

17:28:06 d1 Sinus Rhythm — 70 BPM

25.00 mm/sec 10 mm/mV

this is (not) a circle
a dash – slash – line
tip/fall over it
not/fine/not/fine/not/fine

Tuesday, October 02, 2012 10:32:42

Report Number:

6/14

UBC HOSPITAL
VANCOUVER COASTAL HEALTH

RADIOLOGICAL CONSULTATION

Loc: URAD ACC: [redacted]
Name: [redacted], ELEE
Request MD: BENAVENTE, OSCAR(MD)
Family MD: STANCER, KAREN (MD) L
Age: 42Y F DOB: [redacted]

Exam Date: 18-Jul-2013

CTA

INDICATION: Left vertebral artery dissection for follow-up.

TECHNIQUE: CTA from the arch to the vertex as per CTA stroke protocol.

they escalate
elongate
the hall

control
all the lines
pipe tubes into my skin bag

The intracranial vessels are poorly seen on this study. No gross abnormality of the intracranial arteries is identified. Mild irregularity of the right P1 segment may be due to [redacted]

Cerebral and cerebellar parenchymal appearances are unremarkable given post contrast images. The ventricular configuration is normal and no focal infarct is identified. No extra-axial collection is identified.

IMPRESSION:

she traps a circle of plastic
around my wrist

The appearan ... rtery dissection are
unchanged to ... idence of cerebral or
cerebellar i

unidentity runs
an endless cycle

discomfort, manacle

cut frog silk skin

Last Edited on: 21-Jul-2013 13:32
Reported by: M[redacted] S[redacted] (FEL)
Signed/Proxy by: H[redacted] M[redacted] (MD)
Copy to: T[redacted], JAN(MD)

H[redacted] M[redacted] (MD)
on: 21-Jul-2013 13:32

TRICTLY CONFIDENTIAL - Intended for use of designated recipient only.
If misdirected, or resend desired, fax report with reason to:
604-822-9701 ASAP and destroy this fax immediately.

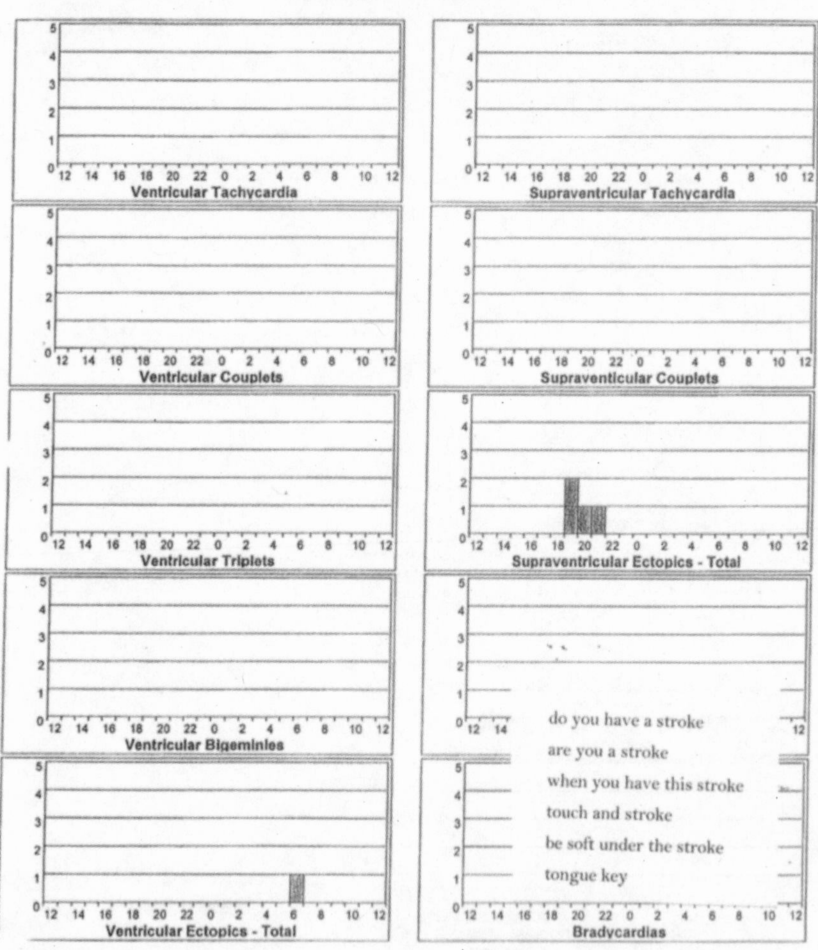

LIFELABS Report Number: [redacted]
Patient: [redacted] ELEE Report Date:10/2/2012 10:19:43 AM

Arrhythmia Histograms

do you have a stroke
are you a stroke
when you have this stroke
touch and stroke
be soft under the stroke
tongue key

Min VT rate: 100 bpm
R on T interval: 370 msec
Min SVE rate: 60 bpm
Pause interval: 2.00 sec
SVE prematurity: 20 %
T wave amplitude: .70 mv
Bradycardia rate: 40 bpm
Blanking period: 250 msec
Bradycardia interval: 300 msec
Form sensitivity: 3

Tuesday, October 02, 2012 10:32:39
Report Number: 78F91C7DC0B2539 2/14

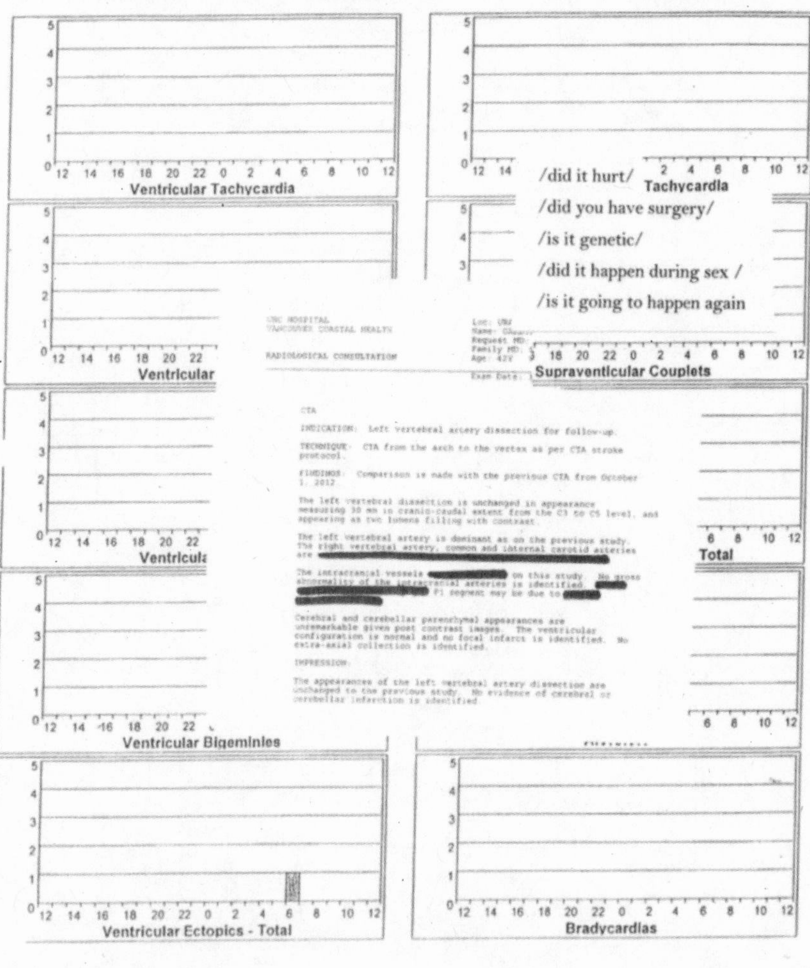

LIFELABS
Patient: , ELEE

Report Number:
Report Date:10/2/2012 10:19:43 AM

Arrhythmia Histograms

/did it hurt/
/did you have surgery/
/is it genetic/
/did it happen during sex /
/is it going to happen again

RADIOLOGICAL CONSULTATION

CTA

INDICATION: Left vertebral artery dissection for follow-up.

TECHNIQUE: CTA from the arch to the vertex as per CTA stroke protocol.

FINDINGS: Comparison is made with the previous CTA from October 1, 2012.

The left vertebral dissection is unchanged in appearance measuring 30 mm in cranio-caudal extent from the C3 to C5 level, and appearing as two lumens filling with contrast.

The left vertebral artery is dominant as on the previous study. The right vertebral artery, common and internal carotid arteries are

The intracranial vessels on this study. No gross abnormality of the intracranial arteries is identified. P1 segment may be due to

Cerebral and cerebellar parenchymal appearances are unremarkable given post contrast images. The ventricular configuration is normal and no focal infarct is identified. No extra-axial collection is identified.

IMPRESSION:

The appearances of the left vertebral artery dissection are unchanged to the previous study. No evidence of cerebral or cerebellar infarction is identified.

Min VT rate: 100 bpm
R on T interval: 370 msec

Min SVE rate: 60 bpm
Pause interval: 2.00 sec

SVE prematurity: 20 %
T wave amplitude: 70 mv

Bradycardia rate: 40 bpm
Blanking period: 250 msec

Bradycardia interval: 300 msec
Form sensitivity: 3

Tuesday, October 02, 2012 10:32:39
2/14

Report Number:

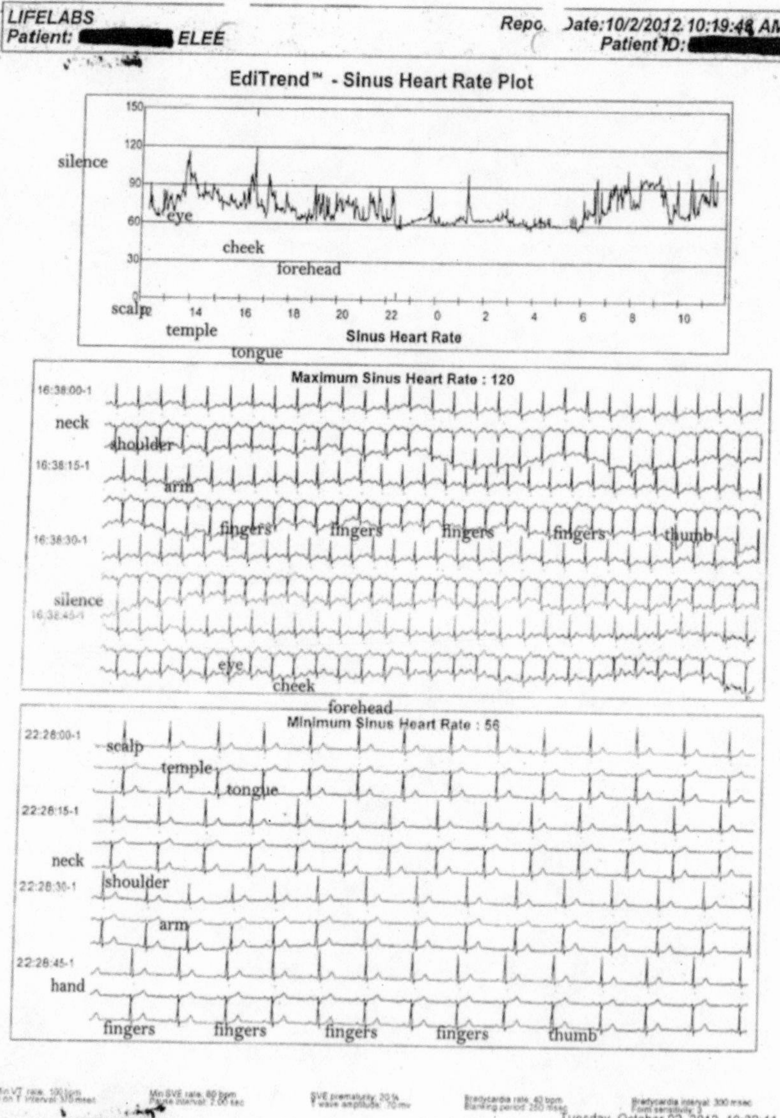

LIFELABS
Patient: ELEE
Date:10/2/2012 10:19:48 AM
Patient ID:
EdiTrend™ - Sinus Heart Rate Plot
silence
eye
cheek
forehead
scalp
temple
tongue
Sinus Heart Rate
Maximum Sinus Heart Rate : 120
16:38:00-1
neck
shoulder
16:38:15-1
arm
fingers
fingers
fingers
fingers
thumb
16:38:30-1
silence
16:38:45-1
eye
cheek
forehead
Minimum Sinus Heart Rate : 56
22:28:00-1
scalp
temple
tongue
22:28:15-1
neck
shoulder
22:28:30-1
arm
22:28:45-1
hand
fingers
fingers
fingers
fingers
thumb
Report Number:
Tuesday, October 02, 2012 10:32:41
3/14

LIFELABS
Patient: [redacted] ELEE

Report Date:10/2/2012 10:19:48 AM
Patient ID:[redacted]

emotional where is chemical lability which response is the sane in an insane situation reflex crying or hormonal or fear-based laughing emotional incontinence pseudobular is it a disorder involuntary emotional expression is it disorder uncontrollable crying – less frequent laughing buzzing neuro blocker oxygen sucker screaming flatlining sweating raging feuding fearing waiting waiting how do I introduce self to me and how long will she be here

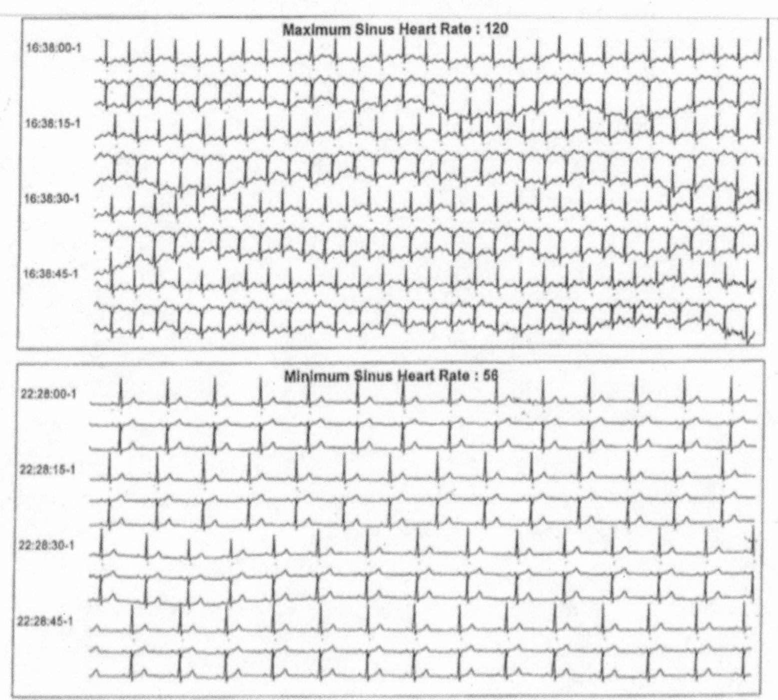

“protect”,”block”,”unblock”,”move”

{“buckets”:{“ignore”:100,”track”:0,”track-front”:0,”track special”:0},”version”:11,”expires”:

[“helpful”,”DESC”],”unhelpful”:[“helpful”,”ASC”],”flagged”:[“age”,”DESC”],”useful”:[“ age”,”DESC”],”resolved”:[“age”,”DESC”],”noaction”:[“age”,”DESC”],”inappropriate”:

:true,”wgEnableWriteAPI”:true,” “wgFormattedNamespaces”:{“-2”:”Media”,”- :false,”skin”:”vector”,”stylepath”:”//bits. org/static-1.23wmf6/skins”,”wgUrlProtocols”

“,[“jquery.fn.focusAt”1”:”Special”,”0”:”“,”1”:”Talk”,”2”:”User”,”3”:”User talk”,”4”:” talk”,”6”:”File”,”7”:”File talk”,”8”:” 9”:” talk”,”108”:”Book”,”109”:”Book talk”,”446”:”

“jquery.util.adaptlettercase .nolanglinks”,”1386876476]
[“ext.eventLogging”]],[“schema.UniversalLanguageSelector”,”1347062400”,[“ext.event Logging”]],[“schema”,”watchlist.schema”,”.schema”,”1347062400,
[“schema.EchoInteraction”,”1347062400”,[“ext.eventLogging”]]]);mw.config.set({“wg LoadScript”:”//bits.wikimedia.org/en.wikipedia.org/load.php”,”debug”

:false,”skin”:”vector”,”stylepath”:”//
skins”,”wgUrlProtocols”:”http\\:\/\/|https\\:\/\/|ftp\\:\/\/|ftps\\:\/\/|ssh\\:\/\/|sftp\\:\/\/|irc\\:\/\/|ircs\\:\/\/|xmpp\\:|sip\\:|sips\\:|gopher\\:\/\/|telnet\\:\/\/|nntp\\:\/\/|world-wind\\:\/\/|mailto\\:|tel\\:|sms\\:|news\\:|svn\\:\/\/|git\\:\/\/|mms\\:\/\/|bitcoin\\:|mag-net\\:|urn\\:|geo\\:|\/\/”,”wgArticlePath”:”/wiki/$1”,”wgScriptPath”:”/w”,”wgScriptEx tension”:”.php”,”wgScript”wgFormattedNamespaces”:{“-2”:”

1”:”Special”,”0”:”“,”1”:”Talk”,”2”:”User”,”3”:”User talk”,”4”:” talk”,”10”:”
12”:”Help”,”13”:”Help talk”,
“14”:”:”Book”,”109”:”Book

talk”,”4461,”“:0,”talk”:1,_talk”:3,”:6,”_talk”:11,”help”:12,”help_talk”:13,”category”:14,”c ategory_talk”:15,” 101,”book”:108,”book_talk”:109,”education_program”:446,”educa-tion_program_talk”:447,”timedtext”:

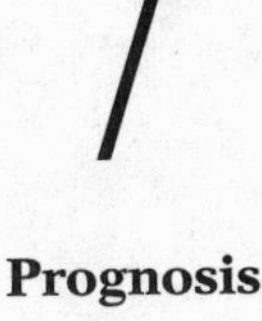

Prognosis

A friend writes about a fig torn open, honeyed drop at the stem. Split skin. Heaviness of tender velvet flesh. Describes the beard of mould this sad fig wore. Her sentences flicker in my head with a curious feeling of pleasure. I turn back to the text perplexed.

Or, within a thing I never liked is the sudden plume of orgasm—a taste of salt or pupilsheen of refrigerated black olives. I bite and feel emotional—either the idea of the olive or the sensation of it trills inside me. I go back to check, try another, spit the pit, roll one on my tongue and the texture lights between thought / memory / sensation.

Thoughtpleasure is also in the memorywhiff of gasoline in the garage. I pull deep and it wanders away. I want the feeling again, in my mind I have this feeling, when I smell it—o, the feeling—a stretch at the base of the spine as I walk up the stairs, idea of delight pressed into body. Cues range: the intake of breath from the confessional Slav smoking on the radio, the taste of frost—these things send me / bring me. Once, the heat of a woman's breath as she leaned over me—I was so close to reaching for her. Everything is erotic: tripwires, switches made of neuroplastic, the pleasure of healing.

Strange how fast we turn corners, start feeling better and forget what we were. For instance, today I biked, broke the glinting spider webs barring the path through the bushes. It is fall, hot and gold, two years gone / gained and I am only aware of this anniversary because of the cycle of time / weather. I went down to the river where the heat coaxed thick, wet fog up from the water. It spumed over the bank as I straddled the bike. I stood still to saturate my lungs with coolness. A seal below me held its silent, compact head above dark water; it breathed with me, its husky exhales a touch. We were waiting for something—the tugboat to pass, the fog to lift. Everything muted gentle as the seal's whiteless eyes. Spoonful by spoonful each day I taste the river, the salt, clouds, all the recipes of blood.

BED: 8 BODY: 40 AWAY: 13 BREATH: 12 DISRUPTION: 9
TEARS: 15 TOUCH: 12 TONGUE: 10 SKIN: 7 LINE: 16

Notes

/ A dissection is a tear within the wall of the artery. In my case, a section of the *tunica intima*, or lining, tore away from the inside of the vertebral artery. Doctors suggest this created the small clot that lodged in my brainstem for a few minutes before dissolving or moving on. As of the last imaging 3.2cm of the *tunica intima* remains unattached and may remain this way without any side effects or dangers.

/ The brain stem controls all basic activities of the central nervous system: consciousness, blood pressure, and breathing. All of the motor control for the body flows through it. Brain stem strokes can impair any or all of these functions and manifest symptoms such as vertigo, dizziness, double vision, slurred speech and decreased level of consciousness. Excerpted and adapted from "Surviving a Brain Stem Stroke," *Stroke Connection*, January/February 2003.

/ The average length of a TIA (transient ischemic attack) is 60 seconds. While TIA is often labeled "mini-stroke," it is more accurately characterized as a "warning stroke." TIA is caused by a clot; the only difference between a stroke and TIA is that with TIA the blockage is transient (temporary) and there are no lingering effects. strokeassociation.org.

/ Each minute stroke treatment is delayed, the average patient loses 1.9 million brain cells, 13.8 billion synapses, and 12 km of axonal fibres. On average, 20% of strokes in patients younger than 45 years of age involve dissections; 50% of patients with vertebral artery dissections experience no neurological deficit; 25% have moderate to severe deficits; 21% experience mild deficits only; 4% of these dissections end in death. From *Canadian Journal of Neurological Sciences*, "Extracranial carotid and vertebral artery dissection: a review," Redekop, G.J., May 2008.

/ In "Psychiatric Issues in Neurology, Part I: Stroke," *Primary Psychiatry*, September 1, 2007, Dr. J. Levenson writes, "Poststroke anxiety may include posttraumatic stress symptoms, anticipatory anxiety about the risk of recurrence, and somatization." Disinhibited and disproportionate laughing and crying are also common.

/ The etiological footnotes gather the incidence of certain words from sections of the text. In medicine, etiology, from the Greek αἰτιολογία meaning "giving a reason for," is the study of causation, why things happen. Etiology can also refer to a myth or origin story. In some ways the writing, which I did in simple, flat lines during the year of healing, narrated the experience back to me once I was well enough to think clearly. Did the condition cause the poem or did the poem create / articulate the conditions of healing? The checklist wording and format are lifted from the medical test requisition forms from my treatment file.

/ Dissections of the extracranial carotid and vertebral arteries arise from tears that occur in the intimal layer, allowing blood under arterial pressure to enter the wall of the vessel and form an intramural hematoma. Disruption of the endothelium can activate platelets and the coagulation cascade, leading to thrombus formation and distal embolization.

The above passage from Redekop's "Extracranial carotid and vertebral artery dissection: a review," was the source text for a series of blind substitutions. As in Mad Libs, I elicited specific parts of speech to fill holes (lumens) I created in the scientific text from angela rawlings, Sikeena Karmali, Nick Flynn, and Christopher Gainey. Some I created myself (false lumens!).

/ Κλωθώ and Ἄτροπος are two of the three Greek fates. The first, Clotho, is the spinner of the thread of life and the latter, Atropos, determines a person's death by cutting the thread with her scissors. The middle sister, Lachesis, measures the length of thread.

/ Both the epigraph and lines I broke into poetic form are from Søren Kierkegaard's *Either/Or, Volume 1*, translated by David F. Swenson and Lillian Marvin Swenson, Princeton University Press, 1971.

/ The line *there is a true and false lumen* is lifted from an angiogram report Oct 1, 2012.

/ The warning: "NOTE: This is information at a point in time and updates/addendums may not be fully reflected on printed copies. The report should be revised again online to ensure the most current information is used before making clinical treatment decisions," is lifted verbatim from a medical file. Although it irks me, I kept intact the use of "addendums" instead of the correct "addenda."

/ I published a chapbook called *Trauma Head* in August 2017 in a limited edition of 50 hand-assembled copies. It was bound as a medical file with the purchaser's choice of three personalized letters on the lip of the file. A few of the poems appear here. I made the chapbook in the waiting time between delivering the manuscript of the long poem "Tunica Intima" and its publication, with the simple goal of keeping my hands busy. The chapbook was manufactured with pages of my medical file, a Sharpie, a photocopier, double-sided tape and scissors.

I was interested in the tension between the high tech visuals in the testing and my low-fi crafting skills.

/ "emotional where is chemical…" integrates the American Heart and Stroke Association's description of pseudobulbar affect with my experience of being emotionally labile post-TIA.

/ « "protect", "block", "unblock", "move" » [sic] uses language from an MRI image of my brain that was created when the video study was converted into an incompatible non-visual computer program.

/ Fig talk in "Prognosis" comes from a beautiful piece of prose by Emiliabianca Pisani.

Acknowledgments

Thank you to those immediately involved in my healing, including Leigh Striegler and everyone at the park that morning; Dr. Oscar Benavente, Franco Cermeno and the Vancouver General Hospital Stroke Prevention Clinic; and Dr. Karen Stancer. Dr. Tenley Albright seamlessly blended medical and emotional care, holding me with the best of current research and the best of mothering. Robert, Beba, and Ivar Kraljii helped make sense of the unexplainable: they are my prime movers, my *mmm* and *ha*, my sweet security. The unceded Musqueam land, the river, the rainforest in which I healed and which heals me: gratitude. Thank you to angela rawlings, whose artistic collaborations gave me a processing mode for this event and whose editorial support has for the second time been a magical and delicious textual friendship. Thank you to the readers who accompanied this recording as it matured from a partial line a day into a book: John Asfour, Alex Leslie, Rachel Patterson, Rachel Rose, Dara-Lyn Shrager and Betsy Warland. Thank you to Nick Flynn, Christopher Gainey, Sikeena Karmali, and angela rawlings for their creative contributions to "enter the disruption." Thank you to Doris Cheung for scans and to Emiliabianca Pisani for figs. Thank you to Jordan Scott and the readers of the chapbook *Trauma Head* who shared their feedback, especially Ali Blythe — and to the ultimate pinecone, angela, for the original idea to make it. Thank you to the 2015 Robert Kroetsch Award for Innovative Poetry and the 2018 bpNichol Chapbook Award for shortlisting versions of this work, and to Daphne Marlatt, Sandra Ridley, and Fred Wah for words of support. To each friend and sister who waited for me to answer, no matter how slowly, thank you.

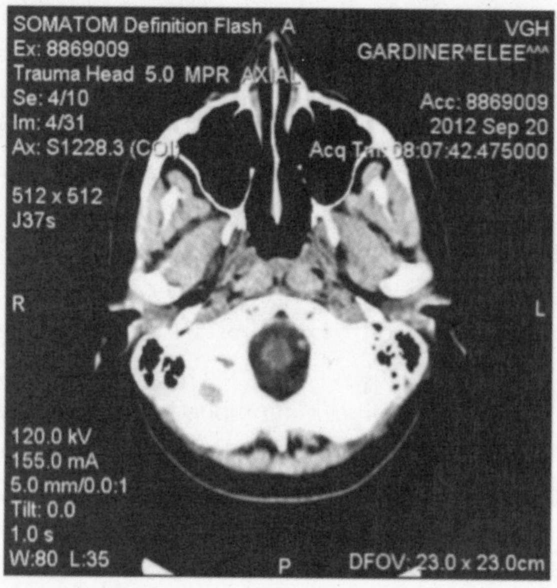

Elee Kraljii Gardiner is the author of *serpentine loop* (Anvil Press, 2016), the co-editor with John Asfour of *V6A: Writing from Vancouver's Downtown Eastside* (Arsenal Pulp Press, 2012), and editor of the forthcoming *Against Death: 35 Essays on Living* (Anvil Press). She was the founder and creative mentor of Thursdays Writing Collective, a non-profit organization of Downtown Eastside writers, and editor and publisher of eight of its anthologies. Originally from Boston, she is a dual US/Canadian citizen. eleekg.com